# WALL PILATES

## *For*

# SENIORS

THE EFFECTIVE 28-DAYS FOR BUILDING STRENGTH, FLEXIBILITY & BALANCE

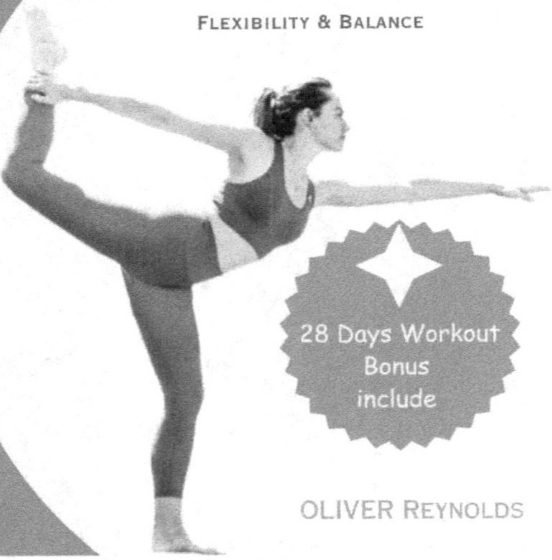

28 Days Workout Bonus include

OLIVER REYNOLDS

# WALL PILATES FOR SENIORS

The Effective 28-Days For Building
Strength, Flexibility & Balance

## Oliver Reynolds

# CONTENTS

# INTRODUCTION

Welcome to a transformative journey that defies age and embraces vitality – "Wall Pilates for Seniors." Within these pages, you will discover a graceful fusion of timeless wisdom and contemporary wellness, designed exclusively for the golden years of life. As we navigate the beautiful tapestry of aging, our bodies yearn for gentle care, vibrant energy, and a renewed sense of purpose. This book is your compass, guiding you towards a healthier, stronger, and more balanced self through the art of Wall Pilates.

In the heart of these chapters lies a treasure trove of insights that celebrate both the wisdom of age and the wonders of movement. Wall Pilates isn't just a fitness routine; it's an ode to the profound synergy between body and mind. With each carefully crafted posture and each intentional breath, you will reconnect with the remarkable resilience of your body and cultivate a harmonious union of strength and grace.

Imagine a life where each morning holds the promise of newfound flexibility, where every step exudes confidence, and where the mirror reflects a vibrant spirit that knows no bounds. "Wall Pilates for Seniors" is your ticket to that reality. From the fundamental principles that govern Wall Pilates to the intricacies of proper alignment and posture, this introduction lays the foundation for your journey towards holistic well-being.

As you turn the pages, be prepared to embark on an exploration of both the physical and the ethereal. Discover how the support of a wall becomes a symbol of your unwavering strength, allowing you to delve into stretches that invigorate your soul. Embrace the delight of each movement that nurtures your core, nourishes your joints, and liberates your spirit. And as your practice unfolds, you will realize that Wall Pilates is not merely a workout; it's an expression of self-love, a sanctuary of rejuvenation, and a testament to age is just a number, after all.

Are you ready to step into a world where wellness knows no bounds? Let "Wall Pilates for Seniors" be your guide, igniting a spark of enthusiasm that transforms your daily routine into a canvas of possibility. Whether you're a novice or a seasoned practitioner, these pages hold the power to elevate your life, redefine your concept of age, and propel you towards a future where every breath is a celebration of the extraordinary journey you've embarked upon.

Turn the page, and let the adventure begin.

## *Why Wall Pilates is Ideal for Seniors*

In the symphony of life, aging is a melody that deserves to be celebrated. And what better way to honor this journey than with Wall Pilates? This unique approach to fitness understands the changing needs of seniors and embraces them with open arms. Unlike intense workout regimens that might feel overwhelming, Wall Pilates extends a gentle invitation to movement that resonates with the rhythms of your body.

The beauty lies in its simplicity. As we age, the walls that once supported us metaphorically take on a new form – they become our partners in movement. The wall becomes an ally, offering stability, support, and a canvas for rejuvenation. Wall Pilates seamlessly marries this supportive structure with tailored exercises that rekindle your strength, flexibility, and overall well-being. By engaging your muscles, enhancing your posture, and honoring your body's unique needs, Wall Pilates offers a pathway to joyous movement that harmonizes with the essence of aging gracefully.

## Benefits of Wall Pilates for Aging Bodies

Embrace the gift of vitality that Wall Pilates brings to your aging body. Beyond the obvious physical advantages, this practice is a transformative journey that honors every milestone your body has achieved. With a focus on gentle, controlled movements, Wall Pilates breathes life into stiff joints, bolsters core strength, and rekindles your connection with balance. It's a dance that fosters mindfulness, creating a symphony of harmony between body, breath, and spirit.

Wall Pilates showers a myriad of benefits upon your aging body. As you lean into the wall's support, you'll notice increased flexibility that not only enhances your range of motion but also alleviates discomfort. Strengthening muscles becomes an act of self-love, creating a shield against the wear and tear of time. With improved posture comes a renewed confidence that radiates from within. And perhaps most importantly, Wall Pilates invites you to partake in a holistic wellness journey that nurtures your mental and emotional well-being, reminding you that age is but a number on the timeline of a life beautifully lived.

## How This Book Can Help You

Welcome to a compass for your journey towards wellness, a guide that transforms Wall Pilates into a life-affirming practice tailored for you. This book isn't just about movements; it's a symphony of guidance, insights, and encouragement meant to accompany you every step of the way. Whether you're a seasoned practitioner or just beginning, this book offers a roadmap to embrace the transformative power of Wall Pilates in your life.

Inside these pages, you'll find clear instructions, illustrated routines, and a wealth of knowledge tailored to seniors. From fundamental principles to advanced postures, each chapter is crafted to empower you, ensuring your practice is both safe and effective. With a 28-day challenge, you're invited to embark on a journey that's not only physical but also mindful – a journey that transcends exercise and becomes a celebration of your spirit's resilience.

Prepare to rediscover the vitality that resides within you. Let this book be your mentor, your companion, and your catalyst for a life enriched by Wall Pilates. Your body deserves this gift, and with this book as your guide, you're poised to unwrap it with joy and gratitude.

# Chapter 1: Understanding Wall Pilates

## *What is Wall Pilates?*

Imagine a canvas where movement is your brushstroke, and the wall is your supporting muse. Welcome to the enchanting world of Wall Pilates, a gentle yet profound approach that melds the wisdom of Pilates with the unwavering support of a wall. At its essence, Wall Pilates is a symphony of controlled movements, breath, and alignment, designed to rejuvenate your body, mind, and spirit. It transforms the wall from an ordinary structure into a guiding force that assists, nurtures, and empowers your journey towards holistic well-being.

In Wall Pilates, the wall becomes more than a mere backdrop; it's a partner in your movement exploration. The wall supports you in poses, offering stability and allowing you to engage with exercises that honor your body's unique needs. By using the wall as an ally, you unlock a realm of possibilities that cater to seniors' specific requirements, ensuring that every stretch, every posture, and every movement resonates deeply with your evolving physicality.

## The Principles of Wall Pilates

At the heart of Wall Pilates lie a set of principles that form the bedrock of this transformative practice. These principles illuminate the path towards effective and mindful movement, shaping a practice that aligns seamlessly with the needs of seniors. Precision, breath, control, and fluidity become your guiding stars, leading you through an orchestrated dance that harmonizes body and soul.

Precision ensures that every movement is intentional, fostering body awareness and rekindling connections that time might have dulled. Breath infuses vitality into each posture, encouraging relaxation and creating a rhythmic flow that energizes your practice. Control empowers you to navigate each movement with grace, instilling a sense of mastery and enhancing your sense of stability. Fluidity merges each motion into the next, allowing you to explore the seamless integration of strength and flexibility.

## *Safety Precautions and Guidelines for Seniors*

Your well-being is paramount, and Wall Pilates embraces this by offering a haven of safe movement. As seniors, your bodies deserve the gentlest care, and this practice understands and caters to those needs. Before you embark on your journey, consider a few essential safety precautions and guidelines that will accompany you throughout your practice.

Start with self-awareness. Listen to your body's cues, acknowledging its limits and its potential. It's advisable to consult your healthcare provider before beginning any new exercise regimen. As you delve into Wall Pilates, honor the principle of gradual progression. Begin with basic postures, gradually building strength and flexibility over time. The wall offers support, but it's essential to maintain proper alignment to prevent strain.

Stay attuned to your breath, letting it be your constant companion as you move. This practice is about mindful movement, not forceful exertion. If any movement causes discomfort or pain, modify or discontinue it.

Remember, your practice is uniquely yours, and it's a journey of self-care and self-discovery.

With these safety precautions and guidelines as your North Star, you're ready to immerse yourself in the enchanting world of Wall Pilates, where every pose becomes a testament to your body's resilience and your spirit's boundless capacity for renewal.

# Chapter 2: The Foundations of Wall Pilates

## *Basic Wall Pilates Techniques and Positions*

Discover the poetry of movement as you embark on the journey of Basic Wall Pilates Techniques and Positions. In this chapter, you'll uncover a palette of poses that seamlessly blend the simplicity of the wall with the elegance of Pilates. These foundational techniques are the cornerstone of your practice, guiding you through a world where the wall becomes your gentle partner in rejuvenation.

Experience the magic of wall-assisted stretches that gently unfold your body's knots, releasing tension like pages of a well-worn book. Engage in leg lifts and squats that enhance strength, bolstering your confidence with every repetition. Feel the exquisite balance of poses like "Wall Tree" and "Wall Warrior," where the wall serves as your constant anchor, reminding you of the stability within and around you. Each posture is a step on the path to rediscovering the grace and flexibility that have always resided within you.

## *Importance of Proper Alignment and Posture*

Alignment and posture are the brushstrokes that paint the masterpiece of your Wall Pilates practice. Imagine your body as a canvas, and each movement as a stroke that, when guided by proper alignment, creates a symphony of grace. This chapter delves into the art of positioning your body in a way that maximizes the benefits of Wall Pilates while safeguarding against strain or injury.

When alignment becomes your compass, you'll find that each movement not only engages specific muscles but also fosters a harmonious connection between body segments. With proper posture, you unveil a canvas of stability that allows you to explore your body's potential with confidence. Aligning your spine, hips, and limbs in sync is the key to unlocking your innate strength, promoting ease of movement, and nurturing a poised stance that echoes your spirit's resilience.

## Breathing Techniques for Effective Wall Pilates

The rhythm of breath is the undercurrent that carries you through the voyage of effective Wall Pilates. In this chapter, you'll learn to embrace the dance of breath, intertwining it with movement to create a symphony that enhances both physical and mental well-being. Breathing techniques are the threads that weave mindfulness into your practice, infusing it with intention and purpose.

Breath is your guide as you glide through poses, reminding you to inhale space and exhale tension. It's the silent whisper that encourages you to explore your limits while respecting your body's boundaries. The art of synchronizing breath with movement transforms your practice into a moving meditation, where each inhale brings clarity and each exhale releases stagnation. Whether you're lengthening your spine against the wall or deepening a stretch, the cadence of your breath creates a bridge between the conscious and the physical, infusing each posture with intention and grace.

As you embrace these techniques, alignment, and breathing, you'll find that Basic Wall Pilates transcends the realm of exercise, becoming a mindful journey that elevates your entire being. Each technique, each alignment, and each breath is a brushstroke that adds depth and vibrancy to the canvas of your practice, creating a masterpiece of movement that speaks volumes about your commitment to holistic wellness.

# **Chapter 3:** Wall Pilates Exercises for Mobility and Flexibility

## *Gentle Neck and Shoulder Stretches*

Welcome to a sanctuary of relief and relaxation, where the gentle embrace of Neck and Shoulder Stretches becomes a balm for the stresses of everyday life. In this chapter, you'll discover a series of movements that honor the intricate interplay of your neck and shoulder muscles. These stretches are more than just physical; they're a symphony of release, easing tension and inviting a soothing sense of calm.

Begin with the simple elegance of neck tilts and rolls, feeling the subtle stretch that unfurls with each movement. Transition to shoulder shrugs that gracefully unravel knots, leaving behind a canvas of renewed vitality. "Wall Neck Stretch" and "Shoulder Opener" positions invite you to lean into the wall's support, allowing your muscles to unwind and your spirit to find serenity. Each stretch is an opportunity to reconnect with your body, inviting a sense of space and relief that resonates deeply.

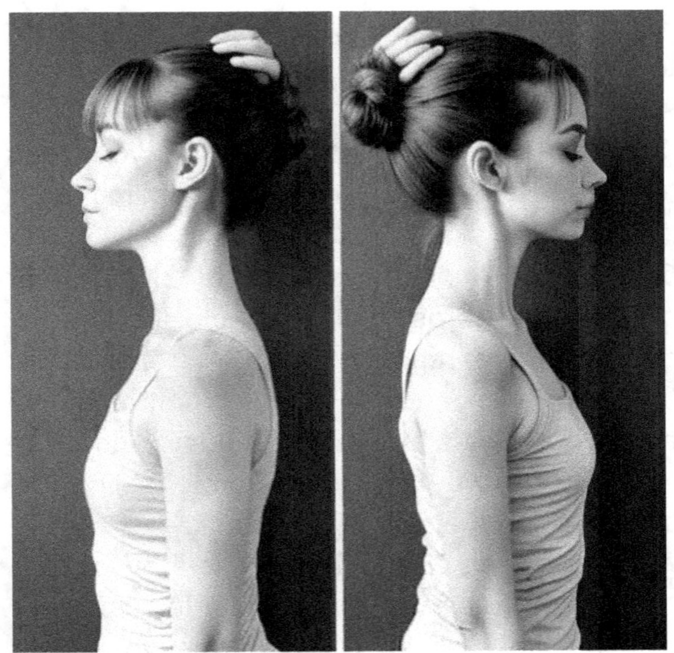

**Practice Guide for Gentle Neck and Shoulder Stretches:**

1. Find a quiet, comfortable space near the wall.

2. Stand with your feet hip-width apart and gently press your back against the wall.

3. Start with gentle neck tilts, moving your ear towards your shoulder and holding for 15-20 seconds on each side.

4. Progress to neck rolls, moving your chin towards your chest and slowly rolling your head to each side.

5. Perform shoulder shrugs by lifting your shoulders towards your ears and then gently dropping them, repeating for 10-15 reps.

6. Experience the "Wall Neck Stretch" by pressing your palm against the wall and tilting your head away from the hand, feeling the stretch along the side of your neck.

7. Practice the "Shoulder Opener" by placing one hand on the wall at shoulder level, fingers pointing behind you. Slowly rotate your torso away from the wall, feeling a gentle stretch in your shoulder and chest.

## Spine Mobility Exercises

Unveil the poetry of your spine's flexibility as you delve into the realm of Spine Mobility Exercises. This chapter invites you to unlock the fluid grace that resides within your vertebrae, creating a harmonious dance between strength and flexibility. With each movement, you'll be guided towards a spine that sways like a willow, adapting to life's rhythms with newfound agility.

Explore cat-cow stretches that flow like a tranquil river, arching and rounding your spine in a graceful sequence. Embrace the "Wall Roll Down," where you articulate your spine vertebrae by vertebrae, releasing any stiffness along the way. 'Spinal Twist ' and 'Seated Forward Fold ' positions take you through twists and bends that honor your body's unique needs, promoting suppleness and fostering a profound sense of liberation.

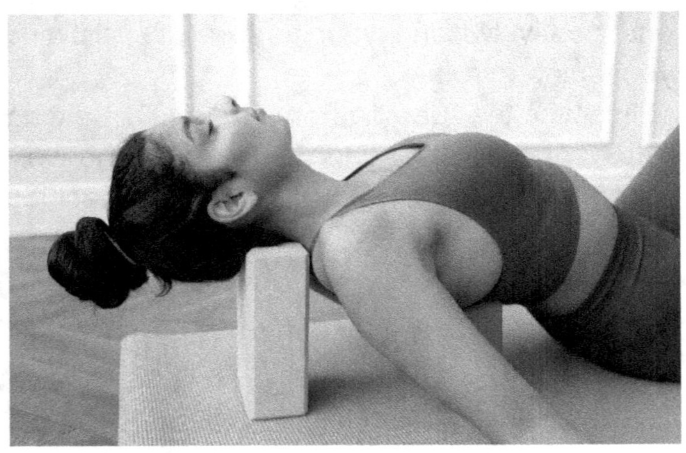

**Practice Guide for Spine Mobility Exercises:**

1. Begin in a comfortable standing position facing the wall.

2. Perform cat-cow stretches by inhaling and arching your back, lifting your chest and tailbone towards the wall. Exhale and round your spine, tucking your chin towards your chest.

3. Experience the "Wall Roll Down" by placing your palms on the wall and slowly rolling down, segment by segment, feeling each vertebra release and lengthen.

4. Engage in the "Spinal Twist" by standing parallel to the wall, placing one hand against it and gently twisting your torso away, allowing your spine to rotate.

5. Practice the "Seated Forward Fold" by sitting with your legs extended, feet against the wall. Hinge at your hips and fold forward, reaching for your feet or ankles.

## *Leg and Hip Flexibility Routines*

The chapters of life are woven through the grace of movement, and Leg and Hip Flexibility

Routines offer a harmonious narrative. This chapter invites you to embrace the canvas of your lower body with stretches that celebrate the majesty of your legs and the resilience of your hips. These routines are a tribute to the fluidity that resides within, guiding you towards a realm of grace and comfort.

Begin with "Wall Quad Stretch," a pose that opens your hip flexors and thighs, promoting both flexibility and balance. Transition to "Hamstring Stretch," where the wall supports your leg as you unfold your hamstring with gentle intent. "Wall Pigeon" and "Seated Butterfly" positions delve into deeper stretches, inviting your hips to release tension and inviting a sense of liberation. Each routine is a step towards reclaiming the ease of movement that echoes the vibrancy of youth.

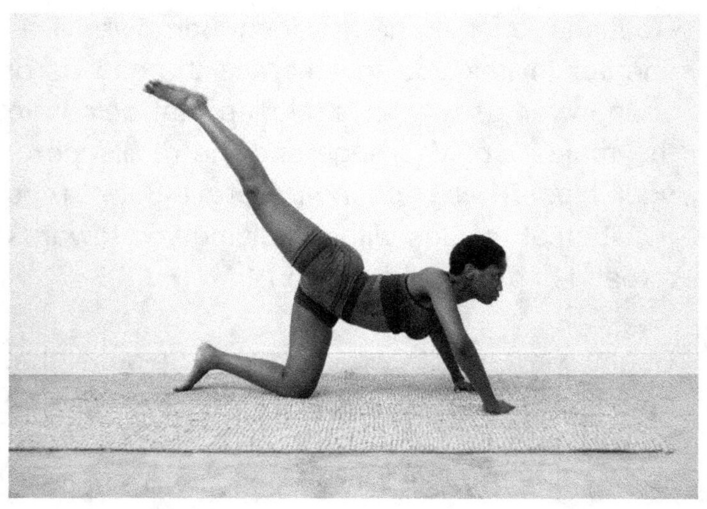

**Practice Guide for Leg and Hip Flexibility Routines:**

1. Stand facing the wall at arm's length.

2. Perform the "Wall Quad Stretch" by bending one knee and grabbing your ankle behind you. Gently press your foot into your hand while keeping your knee pointing down.

3. Experience the "Hamstring Stretch" by lying on your back with one leg extended against the wall. Lift the other leg towards the ceiling, gently pressing it against the wall while keeping your knee straight.

4. Engage in the "Wall Pigeon" by placing one foot against the wall, knee bent at a 90-degree angle. Extend the other leg behind you, feeling a stretch in your hip and glutes.
5. Practice the "Seated Butterfly" by sitting on the floor facing the wall. Press the soles of your feet together and gently push your knees towards the wall, feeling a stretch in your hips and inner thighs.

Each movement in these routines is an ode to the body's exquisite capacity for transformation. By immersing yourself in these practices, you'll rediscover a vitality that transcends age, nurturing flexibility that echoes the vibrant dance of life itself.

# Chapter 4: Building Strength and Stability

## *Core Strengthening Workouts*

Unveil the core's hidden power with the enchanting world of Core Strengthening Workouts. In this chapter, you'll delve into a realm that goes beyond mere exercises – it's a journey of empowerment and self-discovery. These workouts are more than just crunches; they're a symphony of movements that sculpt and strengthen your core, fostering not only physical prowess but also a newfound connection with your body's center.

Experience the grace of "Wall Planks," where the wall becomes your stabilizing force, allowing you to engage your core without the strain. Transition to "Leg Lifts with Wall Support," a movement that elevates leg strength while respecting your body's limits. "Abdominal Twists" and "Side Plank with Wall Assistance" invite you to explore the intricate dance of oblique muscles, creating a canvas of balance and endurance that supports your every move.

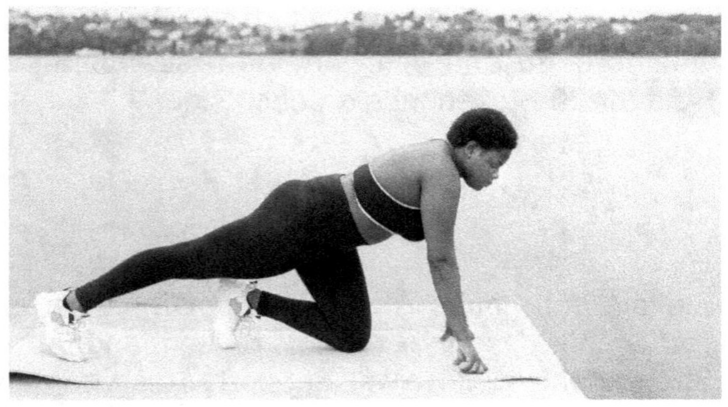

## *Practice Guide for Core Strengthening Workouts:*

1. Begin with "Wall Planks" by placing your forearms on the wall, elbows under your shoulders, and toes on the floor. Maintain a straight line from head to heels, engaging your core. Hold for 20-30 seconds.
2. Engage in "Leg Lifts with Wall Support" by lying on your back with legs extended against the wall. Lift one leg towards the ceiling, engaging your core, and lower it without touching the ground. Repeat for 10-15 reps on each side.
3. Explore "Abdominal Twists" by sitting with your back against the wall, knees bent. Lift your feet off the floor, balancing on your sit bones. Twist your torso to one side and then the other, engaging your obliques.
4. Practice "Side Plank with Wall Assistance" by lying on your side with your legs extended

and feet against the wall. Lift your body onto your forearm and feet, forming a straight line. Hold for 20-30 seconds on each side.

## Leg and Arm Strengthening with Wall Support

Elevate your limbs' strength to new heights as you embark on the journey of Leg and Arm Strengthening with Wall Support. This chapter invites you to discover a symphony of movements that honor both the grace and power of your legs and arms. These strengthening exercises are a testament to the extraordinary potential that lies within, inviting you to cultivate resilience and celebrate the gift of movement.

Begin with "Wall Sit," a pose that fuses leg strength with endurance, allowing you to engage your quadriceps in a stabilizing stance. Transition to "Wall Push-Ups," a movement that elevates your arm strength while providing the support of the wall. "Leg Raises with Wall Support" and "Wall Tricep Dips" delve into a realm of controlled motion, fostering not only strength but also the exquisite art of muscle engagement.

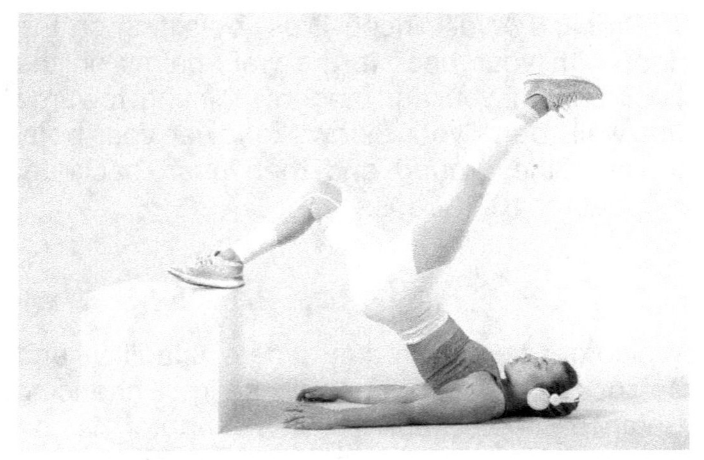

**Practice Guide for Leg and Arm Strengthening with Wall Support:**

1. Begin with "Wall Sit" by leaning your back against the wall and bending your knees, creating a seated position. Hold for 30-60 seconds, engaging your quadriceps.

2. Engage in "Wall Push-Ups" by placing your hands on the wall at shoulder height. Step back and align your body. Lower your chest towards the wall and push back up. Repeat for 10-15 reps.

3. Explore "Leg Raises with Wall Support" by lying on your back with legs extended against the wall. Lift one leg towards the ceiling while keeping the other against the wall. Lower it without touching the floor. Repeat for 10-15 reps on each side.

4. Practice "Wall Tricep Dips" by sitting on the floor with your back to the wall, palms on the floor behind you and fingers pointing towards the wall. Bend your elbows to lower your body towards the ground and then push back up. Repeat for 10-15 reps.

## Enhancing Balance and Stability

Welcome to the realm where stability and balance become your allies in Enhancing Balance and Stability. This chapter is an invitation to cultivate a profound connection with your body's equilibrium, fostering not only physical strength but also mental focus. These exercises are a celebration of poise, a symphony of movements that infuse your steps with grace and your posture with newfound confidence.

Begin with "One-Legged Balance with Wall Touch," a pose that intertwines balance with proprioception, training your body to find steadiness in motion. Transition to "Wall Leg Swings," a movement that elevates lower body flexibility while enhancing your ability to find equilibrium. "Tree Pose with Wall Assistance" and "Chair Pose with Wall Support" delve into a world of mindful balance, creating a canvas where strength and stability harmonize.

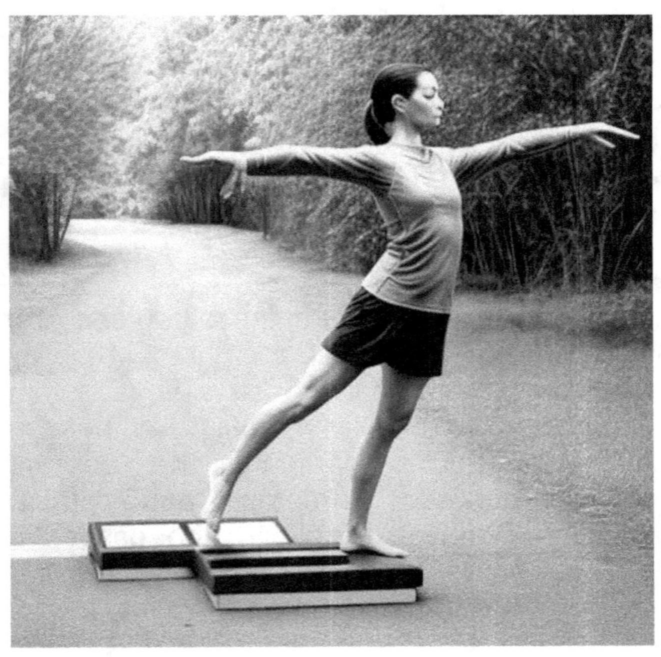

**Practice Guide for Enhancing Balance and Stability**:

1. Start with "One-Legged Balance with Wall Touch" by standing near the wall and lifting one leg. Gently touch the wall for support if needed and hold for 20-30 seconds on each leg.

2. Engage in "Wall Leg Swings" by standing parallel to the wall and using it for support. Swing one leg forward and backward in a controlled motion, feeling a gentle stretch and enhancing balance. Repeat for 10-15 swings on each leg.

3. Explore "Tree Pose with Wall Assistance" by standing with one foot against the wall, placing the sole of the other foot against your inner

thigh. Find your balance and hold for 20-30 seconds on each side.
4. Practice "Chair Pose with Wall Support" by standing facing the wall, a few inches away. Sit back into an imaginary chair, reaching your arms towards the wall for support. Hold for 20-30 seconds.

As you immerse yourself in these Leg and Arm Strengthening and Balance and Stability routines, you're embarking on a voyage that celebrates your body's versatility. With each movement, you're nurturing the delicate balance between strength and grace, cultivating a sense of resilience that echoes in each step you take.

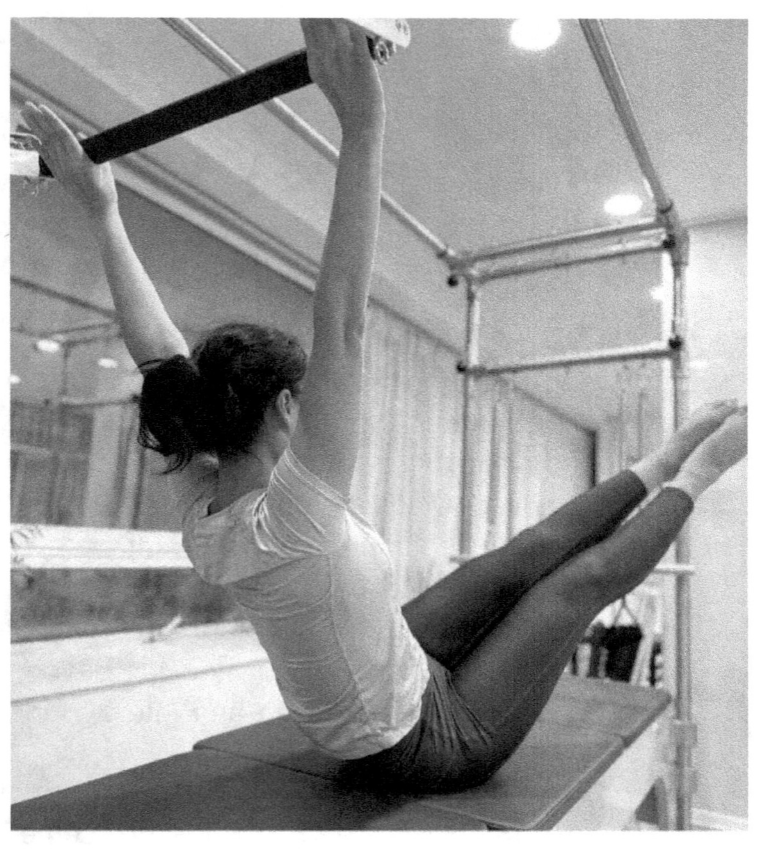

# **Chapter 5**: Relaxation and Mindfulness through Wall Pilates

## *Adding meditation to wall-based Pilates*

By fusing the principles of mindfulness with the art of movement, you can take your Wall Pilates practice to a new level. The chapter "Incorporating Meditation into Wall Pilates" describes a comprehensive method of wellbeing where the balance of the body and mind are intertwined. You'll start a journey of self-awareness via this fusion, moving beyond the scope of simple exercise and into a world of deep connection.

Take a few slow, deep breaths to center yourself and let your breath serve as the link between activity and quiet. Concentrate on the feelings in your body, the pattern of your breath, and the here and now while you do Wall Pilates positions. Feel the firmness of the wall as a reminder of your own steadiness, grounding your ideas and encounters. Each asana, from "Wall Cat-Cow" to "Wall Downward Dog," serves as a blank canvas for meditation, creating a calm environment that enhances your practice.

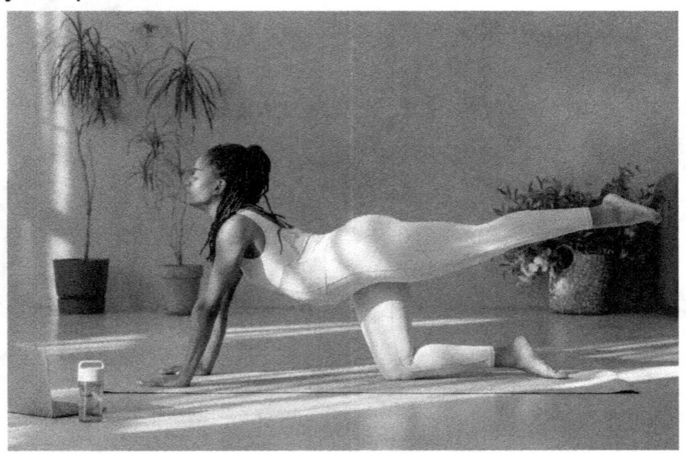

**A Practice Guide for Integrating Meditation into Wall Pilates:**

1. Locate a quiet area next to a wall.

2. To start, take a few minutes to practice deep breathing through your nose.

3. Begin your Wall Pilates routine by paying attention to your body's feelings, your posture's alignment, and the beat of your breath.

4. While doing "Wall Cat-Cow," breathe in as you arch and exhale as you circle your spine.

5. While doing "Wall Downward Dog," keep your breathing steady and feel the stretch in your hamstrings and spine.

6. Accept "Wall Tree Pose" as a moment of attentive balancing, paying attention to the wall's support and your foot's grounding.

7. As you stretch out in "Wall Child's Pose," breathe deeply while experiencing the wall's reassuring presence.

8. Finish your session with a few minutes of sitting meditation, concentrating on your breath and the inner peace.

## Restorative Poses on the Wall

Experience the soft embrace of repair as you learn the skill of "Using the Wall for Restorative Poses." This chapter encourages you to relax into peaceful times and allow the wall to hold you while you refuel physically and mentally. Through these positions, the wall becomes your companion in relaxation, helping you create a haven of silence among the hectic pace of daily life.

Start with the "Supported Legs-Up-the-Wall Pose," a movement that eases stress and promotes tranquility. Go into "Wall Supported Savasana," where the support of the wall acts as a conduit for profound relaxation. Your body needs moderate stretching, therefore "Wall Reclining Butterfly" and "Wall Bridge Pose" lead you into such stretches. Every posture is a call to let go, to rest in the embrace of the wall, and to cultivate a state of being that reflects the rhythm of calm.

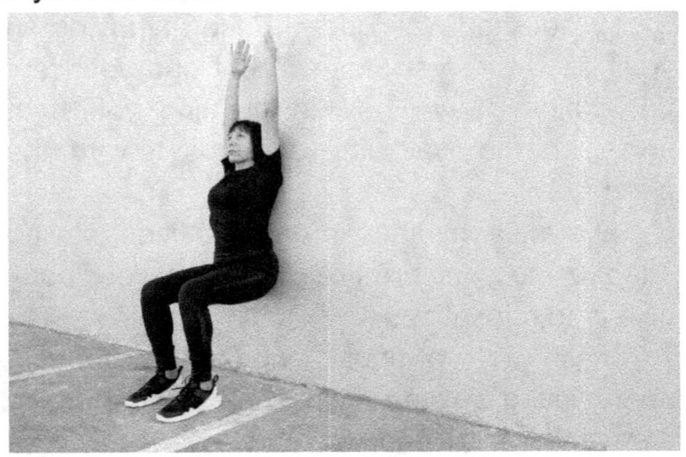

***Practice Guide for Restorative Poses on the Wall:***

1. Make a tranquil area next to the wall.

2. To begin, lean sideways against the wall in the "Supported Legs-Up-the-Wall Pose" before reclining on your back with your legs propped up against the wall. For comfort, place a folded blanket or pillow beneath your hips.

3. Extend your legs up the wall while in "Wall Supported Savasana" while resting on your back. Allow your body to unwind into the support of the wall as you rest your arms at your sides.

4. Sit with your feet together, facing the wall, and slowly let your knees sag to the sides as you embrace "Wall Reclining Butterfly". Your legs should follow the support of the wall.

5. Try out the "Wall Bridge Pose" by laying on your back with your knees bent and your feet up against a wall. While planting your feet firmly on the wall, lift your hips toward the ceiling.

6. Take a few minutes in each position, paying attention to your breath and letting your body give in to relaxation.

7. Finish with a brief period of awareness, appreciating the feeling of renewal and peace that the wall-supported restorative postures have brought.

## Obtaining General Well-Being

As you make your way through the last chapter of your trip, "Achieving Overall Well-being," you will emerge as a well-being masterwork. The spirit of Wall Pilates is captured in this chapter, which goes beyond simple physical exercise to celebrate total wellness. You'll learn how to weave together every aspect of your being into a tapestry of well-being via the beautiful symphony of movement, breath, and awareness.

You are constructing a life that is vibrant and harmonious with each position, each breath, and each attentive moment. The structure of the wall serves as a symbol for the connection between your emotional, mental, and physical selves. You are developing strength and flexibility while you practice Wall Pilates, soothing your mind, and appreciating the beautiful dance of balance.

Allow the effects of your practice to extend beyond the mat and infuse greater awareness into your everyday life. The Wall Pilates principles become your compass, pointing you in the direction of deliberate breathing, correct alignment, and mindful movement not only during your practice but in every action you do. By "Achieving Overall Well-being," you are adopting a way of life that unconditionally loves and cares for your body, mind, and soul, not just a kind of Wall Pilates.

*Here We Go!*

# 28-Day Wall Pilates Challenge

## Week 1: *Foundation Building*

### Day 1-7: Establishing Proper Form and Alignment

**Day 1:** Wall Alignment Check
- Stand facing the wall with heels, hips, and shoulders touching it.
- Align your spine against the wall and ensure your head isn't tilting forward or backward.
- Hold for 1-2 minutes, focusing on maintaining proper posture.

**Day 2:** Wall Squats
- Stand facing the wall, feet hip-width apart.
- Slowly lower into a squat while keeping your back against the wall.
- Push through your heels to return to the starting position.
- Repeat for 10-15 reps.

**Day 3:** Wall Cat-Cow

- Place your hands on the wall, shoulder-width apart.
- Inhale, arch your back, and lift your chest (cow position).
- Exhale, round your back, and tuck your chin (cat position).
- Repeat for 10-12 rounds.

**Day 4:** Wall Planks

- Place your forearms on the wall, elbows under shoulders.
- Step back to create a straight line from head to heels.
- Hold for 20-30 seconds, engaging your core.

**Day 5:** Wall Roll Down

- Stand with your back against the wall, heels a few inches away.
- Roll down, segment by segment, until your back is flat against the wall.
- Roll back up to the starting position.
- Repeat for 8-10 reps.

**Day 6:** Wall Neck Stretch

- Stand with one arm extended against the wall.
- Tilt your head away from the wall, feeling a stretch along the side of your neck.

- Hold for 20-30 seconds on each side.

**Day 7**: **Rest Day**
- Allow your body to recover and prepare for the next week.

# Week 2: *Mobility and Flexibility*

**Day 8-14**: **Improving Joint Mobility and Flexibility**

**Day 8**: **Shoulder Rolls**
- Stand with arms relaxed at your sides.
- Roll your shoulders forward and then backward in controlled circles.
- Repeat for 10-12 rounds in each direction.

**Day 9**: **Wall Leg Swings**
- Stand parallel to the wall, using it for support.
- Swing one leg forward and backward, gently stretching your hamstrings.
- Repeat for 10-15 swings on each leg.

**Day 10**: **Wall Downward Dog**
- Place your hands on the wall at shoulder height.

- Step back and align your body in an inverted "V" shape.
- Press your hips towards the wall, feeling a stretch along your spine.
- Hold for 20-30 seconds.

## Day 11: Wall Reclining Butterfly

- Sit facing the wall with the soles of your feet together.
- Gently let your knees fall to the sides, using the wall for support.
- Hold for 20-30 seconds.

## Day 12: Wall Quad Stretch

- Stand near the wall and grab one ankle behind you.
- Gently press your foot into your hand, feeling a stretch in your quadriceps.
- Hold for 20-30 seconds on each side.

## Day 13: Wall Supported Savasana

- Lie on your back with your legs extended up the wall.
- Rest your arms by your sides and close your eyes.
- Relax and breathe deeply for 5-10 minutes.

## Day 14: Wall Bridge Pose

Lie on your back with your feet against the wall and knees bent.

Press through your feet to lift your hips towards the ceiling.

Keep your arms relaxed by your sides and engage your glutes.

Hold for 20-30 seconds, focusing on your breath and the stretch in your chest and hip flexors.

# Week 3: *Strength and Stability*

**Day 15-21: Progressive Strength-Building Routines with Wall Support**

**Day 15: Wall Push-Ups**
- Stand facing the wall with your hands at shoulder height.
- Step back and align your body in a diagonal line.
- Perform push-ups against the wall for 10-12 reps.

**Day 16: Wall Leg Raises**
- Lie on your back with legs extended against the wall.

- Lift one leg towards the ceiling while keeping the other against the wall.
- Lower it without touching the floor. Repeat for 10-15 reps on each side.

**Day 17**: **Wall Tricep Dips**
- Sit on the floor with your back to the wall, palms on the floor behind you.
- Bend your elbows to lower your body towards the ground.
- Push back up for 10-12 reps.

**Day 18: Wall Plank Variations**
- Perform traditional wall planks (forearms on wall) for 20-30 seconds.
- Then transition to side wall planks, engaging oblique muscles.
- Hold each side plank for 15-20 seconds.

**Day 19: Wall Squat Holds**
- Perform wall squats, lowering into a squat position.
- Hold the squat position for 20-30 seconds.
- Repeat for 3 sets.

**Day 20**: **Wall Supported Single-Leg Stance**
- Stand near the wall and lift one leg off the ground.

- Use the wall for support as you balance on one leg.
- Hold for 20-30 seconds on each leg.

**Day 21**: Rest Day
- Allow your body to recover and prepare for the final week.

# Week 4: *Mind-Body Connection*

**Day 22-28: Combining Relaxation Techniques and Pilates for Holistic Well-being**

**Day 22**: Wall Meditation
- Find a comfortable seated position near the wall.
- Close your eyes, focus on your breath, and let go of tension.
- Meditate for 5-10 minutes.

**Day 23**: Mindful Wall Planks
- Perform wall planks with a focus on breath awareness.
- Inhale as you lower your body and exhale as you push back up.
- Repeat for 10-12 reps.

**Day 24:** Wall Restorative Poses
- Practice "Supported Legs-Up-the-Wall Pose" and "Wall Reclining Butterfly."
- Allow the wall to support you in these restorative stretches.

**Day 25:** Pilates Flow with Wall Assistance
- Create a flow combining wall-assisted poses.
- Move mindfully, focusing on your breath and alignment.

**Day 26:** Wall Savasana
- Lie on your back with legs extended up the wall.
- Close your eyes and relax, letting go of stress.
- Enjoy a deep relaxation for 10-15 minutes.

**Day 27:** Wall Guided Visualization
- Sit or lie down facing the wall.
- Close your eyes and visualize a serene, peaceful place.
- Let your imagination transport you to a tranquil setting.

**Day 28:** Completion and Reflection
- Reflect on your 28-day journey of Wall Pilates.

- Write down your insights, progress, and how you feel.
- Celebrate your commitment to holistic well-being.

Congratulations on completing the 28-Day Wall Pilates Challenge! By progressing through these weekly routines, you've embraced the synergy of movement, mindfulness, and strength. Your body is now more resilient, your mind more focused, and your spirit more aligned with wellness. As you move forward, remember that the principles and practices of Wall Pilates can continue to enrich your life with vitality and harmony.

# CONCLUSION

## Reflecting on Your 28-Day Journey

As you stand at the culmination of your 28-day Wall Pilates journey, take a moment to savor the progress you've made. Each pose, each breath, and each day has woven a tapestry of strength and mindfulness. The commitment you've shown to yourself is a celebration of your well-being's importance. Carry the lessons of alignment, flexibility, and balance into your life, knowing that this journey is not an end but a catalyst for continued growth. The echoes of your dedication resonate within, reminding you that transformation is a constant companion on your path to wellness.

## Continuing Your Wall Pilates Practice

Your 28-day journey through Wall Pilates has illuminated a path of vitality that need not end here. With each movement and breath, you've cultivated a sacred connection between your body and mind. Carry this newfound wisdom forward, letting it infuse every step you take. The wall, once a support, now becomes a reminder of your inner strength. Make Wall Pilates an integral part of your routine, allowing its principles to sculpt not just your body, but also your spirit. With the wall as your ally, your journey of holistic wellness is destined to be an ongoing symphony of health and grace.

## Embracing Lifelong Fitness for Seniors

As you've explored the art of Wall Pilates, you've shattered stereotypes and embraced a truth: fitness is timeless. This 28-day journey is just a glimpse of the boundless potential within you. Remember, age is not a limitation; it's an invitation to nurture your well-being. Your commitment to Wall Pilates is an affirmation that age is but a number, and the pursuit of wellness knows no boundaries. Carry this torch of lifelong fitness with pride, knowing that your dedication is a beacon of inspiration for all. With each day, you're scripting a legacy of vitality that defies expectations and sets a remarkable example for generations to come.